COMPLETE STARCH SOLUTION DIET COOKBOOK RECIPES

A Culinary Journey into Starch-Free Living, Low-Carb Delights, and Transformative Recipes for Weight Loss Success

Norval Ernser

Copyright

Table of contents

Introduction

In the bustling city of Culinary Haven, there lived a young woman named Emily. She was an avid reader, and her small apartment was filled with shelves stacked high with books of all genres. However, her true passion lay in the world of healthy living and nutrition.

One day, as Emily strolled through a local bookstore, a particular book caught her eye – **"The Complete Starch Solution Diet Cookbook Recipes."** Intrigued, she picked it up and flipped through its pages. The vibrant images and enticing descriptions of wholesome, plant-based meals captured her imagination. Without a second thought, Emily purchased the book and headed home.

Little did she know that this impulsive decision would transform her life.

As Emily delved into the pages of the cookbook, she discovered a treasure trove of recipes designed to optimize health through the consumption of plant-based starches. The book outlined a revolutionary approach to nutrition, emphasizing the benefits of whole foods, particularly those rich in complex carbohydrates.

Armed with the knowledge gleaned from the book, Emily embarked on a culinary adventure. She meticulously followed the recipes, experimented with flavors, and discovered the joy of creating delicious meals that also nourished her body. The kitchen became her haven, and the aroma of wholesome ingredients filled the air.

Word of Emily's newfound culinary prowess spread through Culinary Haven like wildfire. Friends and neighbors marveled at her vibrant energy and radiant glow. Intrigued by her transformation, they flocked to her for advice on how to achieve a healthier lifestyle.

Emily, fueled by her passion for sharing the benefits of the Complete Starch Solution Diet, started hosting cooking workshops in her apartment. The small space soon transformed into a bustling hub of culinary creativity, as people from all walks of life gathered to learn and savor the delights of plant-based eating.

As the community around Emily grew, so did her influence. She became a local wellness icon, and her story even caught the attention of a renowned health and wellness magazine. They featured her in an article, highlighting her journey from a simple book purchase to becoming a beacon of health and inspiration in Culinary Haven.

Emily's journey was a testament to the transformative power of knowledge and the impact one person could have on an entire community. The Complete Starch Solution Diet Cookbook became not just a collection of recipes for her, but a guidebook that led her to a life filled with purpose and well-being. And so, in the heart of Culinary Haven, Emily continued to spread the joy of healthy living, one plant-based meal at a time.

Chapter 1: Embracing Starch-Free Living

In the vibrant landscape of dietary choices, the path to optimal health often leads us to unexpected territories. In this chapter, we embark on a transformative journey into the realm of Starch-Free Living, a paradigm shift that promises not only improved well-being but also a sustainable approach to shedding unwanted weight.

Introduction to Starch-Free Living

Let's begin by unraveling the essence of Starch-Free Living. Delve into the core principles that define this lifestyle, understanding the role starch plays in our daily diet and the profound impact its exclusion can have on our health. Discover how this choice extends beyond a mere culinary decision to become a holistic approach to nurturing your body.

Understanding the Health Benefits

The allure of Starch-Free Living lies not only in what it eliminates but also in the vast array of health benefits it introduces. Uncover the science behind this choice – how it can enhance your energy levels, improve digestion, and potentially alleviate various health concerns. Prepare to be inspired by the compelling reasons to embrace this transformative lifestyle.

Jumpstarting Your Journey to a Healthier You

Embarking on a new dietary path can be both exhilarating and challenging. In this section, we provide you with practical tips and strategies to kickstart your journey into Starch-Free Living. From grocery shopping guidance to meal preparation hacks, equip yourself with the tools needed to seamlessly integrate this lifestyle into your daily routine.

As we navigate the introductory waters of Starch-Free Living, the voyage promises not just a change in eating habits but a holistic transformation that resonates throughout your entire well-being. Get ready to embrace a lifestyle that not only revolutionizes your plate but also revitalizes your health and vitality.

Introduction to Starch-Free Living

Welcome to a transformative journey that goes beyond the ordinary realms of dietary choices – a journey into the heart of Starch-Free Living. In this chapter, we peel back the layers of conventional eating habits to explore a lifestyle that has the potential to redefine your relationship with food and elevate your overall well-being.

Starch, a ubiquitous component of many diets, plays a significant role in our daily meals. However, as we delve into the principles of Starch-Free Living, we challenge the status quo, questioning the impact of this commonly consumed element on our health. This exploration is not just about eliminating starch; it's about understanding the profound effects of this choice on our bodies and minds.

As we navigate this introduction, envision Starch-Free Living as more than a dietary adjustment; it's a holistic approach to nourishment. This lifestyle encourages mindful choices that extend beyond the plate, emphasizing the interconnectedness of nutrition, energy levels, and overall vitality.

Why Starch-Free Living?

Consider the enticing prospect of renewed energy, improved digestion, and a potential avenue for weight management. Starch-Free Living is not merely a departure from the familiar; it is an invitation to discover a vibrant, health-focused way of life. Throughout this chapter, we unfold the compelling reasons to embrace this dietary shift, empowering you with knowledge to make informed choices for a healthier you.

Navigating the Unfamiliar Terrain

Embarking on the Starch-Free Living journey may seem like charting unknown waters. Fear not, as we guide you through the initial steps. From understanding food labels to identifying unexpected sources of starch, we equip you with the insights needed to make confident choices. This introduction is your compass, pointing you toward a path where health and nourishment intertwine seamlessly.

As we embark on this exploration, keep an open mind, and be prepared to witness not just a change in diet but a shift in your perspective on what it means to truly nourish your body. Let the journey into Starch-Free Living begin – a journey that promises not just a transformation of your plate but a revitalization of your health and well-being.

Understanding the Health Benefits

Now that we've opened the door to the world of Starch-Free Living, let's delve deeper into the captivating realm of health benefits that accompany this transformative lifestyle. Beyond the mere exclusion of starch, there lies a rich tapestry of advantages that can significantly impact your well-being.

Unlocking the Energy Reservoir

One of the standout benefits of embracing a Starch-Free Living approach is the potential for a substantial boost in energy levels. Starch, a primary source of carbohydrates, is often linked to fluctuations in energy throughout the day. As we eliminate or reduce starch intake, you may discover a newfound vitality, a sustained energy reservoir that propels you through your daily activities with renewed vigor.

Enhancing Digestive Harmony

Starch-Free Living presents an opportunity to foster digestive well-being. For some individuals, starches can pose challenges to the digestive system, leading to bloating, discomfort, and other digestive issues. By choosing a Starch-Free path, you may experience a more harmonious digestive process, promoting gut health and overall comfort after meals.

The Weight Management Advantage

Many individuals turn to Starch-Free Living as a strategy for weight management. The lifestyle's inherent focus on nutrient-dense, whole foods can contribute to a feeling of fullness, potentially reducing overall caloric intake. Through this chapter, we unravel the connection between starch, metabolism, and weight, providing insights that can aid you in achieving your health and wellness goals.

Potential Health Improvements

Beyond energy, digestion, and weight management, Starch-Free Living has been associated with various health improvements. Individuals have reported positive changes in conditions such as inflammation, skin issues, and hormonal balance. While individual responses may vary, this chapter aims to shed light on the potential broader health benefits that adopting a Starch-Free lifestyle may bring.

As we navigate the intricate web of health benefits associated with Starch-Free Living, consider this chapter as your guide to understanding how a shift in dietary choices can ripple through multiple facets of your well-being. Prepare to be intrigued by the possibilities that lie ahead as you continue to embrace the journey toward a healthier, more vibrant you.

Jumpstarting Your Journey to a Healthier You

Congratulations on taking the initial steps toward Starch-Free Living! As we stand at the threshold of this transformative lifestyle, let's explore the practical aspects and actionable steps that will propel you into a healthier and more vibrant version of yourself.

Setting the Stage: The Starch-Free Pantry

Building a foundation for Starch-Free Living begins with your pantry. In this section, we guide you through the art of stocking a Starch-Free pantry. From essential ingredients to recommended substitutions, we ensure you're well-equipped to embark on this journey without compromising on flavor or variety.

Decoding Food Labels

Navigating the grocery store aisles can be a daunting task, especially when embracing a new dietary approach. We demystify food labels, helping you identify hidden starches and make informed choices. Armed with this knowledge, you'll confidently select foods that align with your Starch-Free goals.

Meal Preparation Hacks: Simple and Delicious

The heart of Starch-Free Living lies in the meals you prepare. This section provides practical tips and time-saving hacks for crafting simple yet delicious Starch-Free meals. From quick breakfast options to satisfying dinner ideas, we aim to make your journey seamless and enjoyable.

Planning for Success: Weekly Meal Plans

Staying committed to a Starch-Free lifestyle is made easier with strategic planning. Discover the art of crafting weekly meal plans tailored to your preferences and schedule. These plans not only save time but also ensure you have a variety of tasty, Starch-Free options at your fingertips.

Embracing the Community: Support and Encouragement

Embarking on any lifestyle change is more enjoyable and sustainable when shared with like-minded individuals. We explore the importance of community support, offering tips on finding Starch-Free recipes, connecting with fellow enthusiasts, and celebrating successes together.

As you absorb the insights and practical guidance in this section, remember that transitioning to Starch-Free Living is a journey, not a race. This chapter serves as your compass, helping you lay a solid foundation for a healthier lifestyle. With your pantry stocked, labels decoded, and meal plans in hand, you're ready to embrace the exciting adventure that lies ahead on the path to a healthier you.

Chapter 2: The Science Behind Starch-Free Diets

Embarking on the Starch-Free Living journey involves more than just changing what's on your plate; it's about understanding the intricate science that underpins this transformative dietary choice. In this chapter, we delve into the fascinating world of the scientific principles behind Starch-Free Diets.

Breaking Down Starch and Its Impact

To comprehend the science of Starch-Free Living, we first need to unravel the complexities of starch itself. We explore the molecular structure of starch, its role in energy production, and how the body processes this carbohydrate. By breaking down the science, you gain insights into why limiting or eliminating starch can lead to profound changes in your overall health.

How Starch-Free Living Boosts Metabolism

Metabolism, the body's intricate energy management system, plays a crucial role in Starch-Free Living. Discover how this dietary approach can influence metabolic processes, potentially enhancing your body's ability to burn calories efficiently. Uncover the mechanisms through which Starch-Free Living may contribute to a more dynamic and responsive metabolism.

Exploring the Connection Between Starch and Weight Loss

Weight management is a common goal for many embracing Starch-Free Living. This section explores the relationship between starch consumption, insulin response, and weight gain. By understanding the intricate dance between these elements, you gain valuable insights into how Starch-Free Living might be a key player in your journey towards achieving and maintaining a healthy weight.

As we navigate the scientific terrain of Starch-Free Diets, prepare to be enlightened by the compelling research and evidence supporting this transformative lifestyle. By the end of this chapter, you'll not only grasp the foundational principles but also appreciate the profound impact that Starch-Free Living can have on your body's intricate processes. Get ready to empower yourself with knowledge as you continue on the path toward a healthier and more vibrant you.

Breaking Down Starch and Its Impact

To embark on a journey of Starch-Free Living is to delve into the intricate world of carbohydrates, with starch standing at the forefront. In this section, we unravel the molecular complexities of starch and explore its profound impact on our bodies.

Understanding the Molecular Structure

At its core, starch is a polysaccharide – a complex chain of glucose molecules intricately linked together. As we consume starchy foods, enzymes in our digestive system begin the process of breaking down these chains into simpler sugars like glucose. This intricate dance within our digestive tract is fundamental to understanding how our bodies derive energy from starch.

Starch as a Primary Energy Source

Historically, starch has been a primary energy source for human civilizations. Its rapid conversion into glucose provides a quick and accessible fuel for our cells. However, the abundance of starch in modern diets, often in processed and refined forms, has led to concerns about its impact on overall health, prompting the exploration of Starch-Free Living as an alternative approach.

The Insulin Response Mechanism

One key aspect of starch metabolism involves the release of insulin, a hormone crucial for regulating blood sugar levels. Starchy foods can cause a spike in blood sugar, triggering an insulin response to shuttle glucose into cells for energy. While this process is essential, the excessive consumption of starch may lead to insulin resistance, a condition associated with various health issues, including weight gain and metabolic dysfunction.

Impact on Blood Sugar Levels

The rapid conversion of starch into glucose can result in fluctuations in blood sugar levels. Frequent spikes and crashes in blood sugar may contribute to feelings of fatigue, cravings, and overeating. Understanding this dynamic provides a foundation for comprehending how a Starch-Free approach may offer a more stable and sustainable energy source for the body.

By breaking down the molecular intricacies of starch and its impact on our metabolic processes, we lay the groundwork for a comprehensive understanding of why individuals are increasingly turning to Starch-Free Living as a means to optimize their health. The journey into Starch-Free Living involves not only a shift in dietary choices but a nuanced comprehension of the science that guides this transformative lifestyle.

How Starch-Free Living Boosts Metabolism

In the intricate dance of metabolic processes, Starch-Free Living emerges as a compelling partner, offering potential benefits that extend beyond dietary preferences. Let's delve into the fascinating science behind how embracing a Starch-Free lifestyle can give your metabolism a boost.

Metabolic Flexibility: Adapting to Starch-Free Living

The cornerstone of Starch-Free Living lies in encouraging metabolic flexibility, the body's ability to efficiently switch between different fuel sources. When starch intake is limited, the body becomes adept at utilizing alternative energy pathways, such as fat metabolism. This adaptability is thought to enhance overall metabolic efficiency and may contribute to improved energy utilization.

Ketosis: A Metabolic Shift

One notable aspect of Starch-Free Living is the potential induction of ketosis. In the absence of abundant carbohydrates, the body begins breaking down fats into ketones, which serve as an alternative fuel source. Ketosis is associated with increased fat burning, providing a metabolic advantage for those seeking weight management and enhanced energy levels.

Balancing Hormones for Metabolic Harmony

Starch-Free Living has been linked to improved insulin sensitivity, a crucial factor in metabolic health. By reducing starch intake, individuals may experience more stable blood sugar levels, leading to a more regulated insulin response. This, in turn, can contribute to better control over hunger and satiety, fostering an environment conducive to weight management.

Caloric Efficiency: A Potential Contributor to Weight Loss

Beyond the metabolic shift towards fat utilization, Starch-Free Living often emphasizes nutrient-dense, whole foods. This not only provides essential vitamins and minerals but can also contribute to a feeling of fullness, potentially leading to a reduction in overall caloric intake. The combination of these factors may play a role in the weight management aspect of Starch-Free Living.

As we navigate the intricate landscape of metabolic processes, it becomes clear that Starch-Free Living isn't just about what you exclude from your diet; it's a strategic choice that can positively impact how your body utilizes and manages energy. By understanding the science behind the metabolic advantages, you gain insights into the potential benefits that await you on the Starch-Free journey toward a healthier, more vibrant metabolism.

Exploring the Connection Between Starch and Weight Loss

In the pursuit of optimal health and well-being, the relationship between dietary choices and weight management is a focal point of interest. In this section, we embark on an exploration of the intricate connection between starch consumption and the potential for weight loss within the context of Starch-Free Living.

Insulin Sensitivity and Fat Storage

One pivotal aspect of the Starch-Free approach is its potential impact on insulin sensitivity. Starchy foods can lead to rapid spikes in blood sugar levels, prompting an insulin response. Over time, repeated surges of insulin can contribute to insulin resistance, a condition associated with increased fat storage, particularly around the abdominal region. By reducing starch intake, individuals may enhance insulin sensitivity, potentially curbing the body's inclination to store excess fat.

Starch, Appetite Regulation, and Satiety

The influence of starch on appetite regulation is a nuanced interplay of hormonal responses. Starchy foods can sometimes lead to fluctuations in blood sugar levels, triggering feelings of hunger shortly after consumption. Starch-Free Living, with its emphasis on nutrient-dense, satiating foods, aims to create a more stable environment for hunger and satiety hormones. This, in turn, may contribute to a more controlled and satisfying eating experience, potentially aiding in weight management efforts.

Caloric Density and Nutrient Content

Starch-Free Living often involves a shift towards whole, nutrient-dense foods that are inherently lower in caloric density. This strategic approach allows individuals to consume satisfying portions while potentially reducing overall caloric intake. By focusing on the quality of nutrients, individuals can nourish their bodies with essential vitamins and minerals without the excess baggage of empty calories.

Metabolic Efficiency and Sustainable Weight Loss

The metabolic adaptations that accompany Starch-Free Living, such as the potential induction of ketosis and improved insulin sensitivity, may create an environment conducive to sustainable weight loss. By tapping into alternative fuel sources and optimizing hormonal balance, individuals adopting a Starch-Free lifestyle may find a holistic approach to achieving and maintaining a healthy weight.

As we unravel the connection between starch and weight loss within the framework of Starch-Free Living, it becomes apparent that this dietary choice is not just about shedding pounds; it's about fostering a metabolic environment that supports long-term well-being. The journey into Starch-Free Living offers a scientific perspective on how your dietary choices can influence the complex interplay of factors that contribute to a healthy weight and a vibrant, energetic life.

Chapter 3: Crafting a Top Low Carb Diet Meal Plan

In the pursuit of a healthier lifestyle, crafting a well-balanced and sustainable low-carb meal plan is a cornerstone of success. This chapter is your guide to designing a top-notch Low Carb Diet Meal Plan that not only aligns with your dietary goals but also brings a variety of flavors and nutrients to your plate.

Building Your Perfect Low Carb Plate

The foundation of a successful Low Carb Diet Meal Plan begins with understanding the components of a balanced plate. In this section, we explore the art of building a low-carb plate that combines essential macronutrients – proteins, fats, and carbohydrates – in a way that supports your health objectives. Discover how to create meals that are not only low in carbohydrates but also rich in nutritional value.

Balancing Macronutrients for Optimal Results

Achieving the right balance of macronutrients is key to the success of a Low Carb Diet Meal Plan. We delve into the significance of proteins, fats, and carbohydrates in your diet, providing insights into how each contributes to overall well-being. Learn how to tailor your macronutrient ratios to meet your specific health goals, whether it be weight management, increased energy, or improved athletic performance.

Tailoring Your Meal Plan to Your Lifestyle

One size does not fit all when it comes to meal planning. In this section, we explore how to tailor your Low Carb Diet Meal Plan to suit your unique lifestyle, preferences, and dietary needs. Whether you're a busy professional, a fitness enthusiast, or a culinary adventurer, we provide practical tips and customizable strategies to ensure your meal plan seamlessly integrates into your daily routine.

Crafting a top Low Carb Diet Meal Plan is not just about restriction; it's an opportunity to explore a world of delicious and satisfying foods that align with your health objectives. As we journey through this chapter, prepare to gain the knowledge and tools needed to create a meal plan that not only supports your low-carb lifestyle but also brings joy to your culinary experience. Get ready to savor the benefits of a thoughtfully crafted Low Carb Diet Meal Plan that fuels your journey towards a healthier and more vibrant you.

Building Your Perfect Low-Carb Plate

The cornerstone of a successful Low Carb Diet Meal Plan lies in the artful construction of a well-balanced plate. In this section, we delve into the fundamental principles of building a low-carb plate that not only caters to your dietary objectives but also invites a symphony of flavors and nutrients to every meal.

The Foundation: Non-Starchy Vegetables

At the heart of your low-carb plate are non-starchy vegetables – vibrant, nutrient-rich, and low in carbohydrates. These form the foundation, providing essential vitamins, minerals, and fiber without the carb-heavy load. Dive into a world of leafy greens, cruciferous vegetables, and colorful peppers as you lay the groundwork for a nourishing and satisfying meal.

Protein Powerhouse: Lean and Flavorful

Building on the vegetable foundation, introduce a generous portion of lean protein. Whether it's grilled chicken, fish, tofu, or legumes, protein is a vital component that promotes satiety and supports muscle health. Explore various cooking methods and seasoning techniques to infuse your protein with delicious flavors, creating a centerpiece that anchors your low-carb plate.

Healthy Fats: The Essential Finishing Touch

Complete your perfect low-carb plate with the incorporation of healthy fats. Avocado slices, olive oil drizzles, or a sprinkle of nuts and seeds add not only richness and flavor but also contribute to a satisfying and satiating meal. Embrace the idea that fats can be a valuable ally in your low-carb journey, providing sustained energy and enhancing the overall enjoyment of your culinary creations.

Balancing Act: Tailoring Portions for Success

Achieving the right balance is key to the success of your low-carb plate. This section guides you on portion control, helping you strike the perfect balance between vegetables, protein, and fats. Understanding the synergy between these components ensures that your meal is not only delicious but also aligned with your health and wellness goals.

As you embark on the journey of building your perfect low-carb plate, embrace the creativity and diversity that this approach to meal planning offers. Let each plate become a canvas where you can express your culinary preferences while staying true to the principles of a low-carb lifestyle. Through thoughtful construction, discover the joy of crafting meals that are not only satisfying but also propel you towards your health and wellness aspirations.

Balancing Macronutrients for Optimal Results

Creating a top-notch Low Carb Diet Meal Plan goes beyond simply reducing carbohydrate intake; it involves a strategic balance of macronutrients to optimize your overall well-being. In this section, we unravel the significance of proteins, fats, and carbohydrates, guiding you to achieve the ideal macronutrient balance for your health goals.

The Importance of Proteins

Proteins play a pivotal role in a low-carb meal plan, contributing to muscle health, satiety, and overall metabolic function. Lean meats, poultry, fish, tofu, and legumes are excellent sources of protein that can be incorporated into your meals. Learn how to calculate your protein needs, ensuring an adequate intake to support your body's daily functions and potential fitness endeavors.

Embracing Healthy Fats

Contrary to traditional notions, fats are not the enemy in a low-carb lifestyle – they are a valuable ally. Healthy fats contribute to sustained energy, aid in the absorption of fat-soluble vitamins, and enhance the flavor and satiety of your meals. Avocados, olive oil, nuts, and seeds are stellar examples of incorporating healthy fats into your low-carb plate. Discover how to strike the right balance to meet your nutritional requirements and personal preferences.

Strategic Carbohydrate Choices

While the focus is on reducing overall carbohydrate intake, selecting the right carbohydrates is equally crucial. Opt for complex, fiber-rich carbs found in non-starchy vegetables, nuts, and seeds. This strategic approach ensures that your low-carb meal plan remains nutrient-dense, providing essential vitamins and minerals without the excessive carb load.

Customizing Ratios for Your Goals

The optimal macronutrient ratio varies based on individual factors such as activity level, metabolism, and health objectives. Whether you're aiming for weight loss, muscle gain, or sustained energy, this section guides you through the process of customizing your macronutrient ratios. Understanding the unique needs of your body allows you to tailor your low-carb meal plan for optimal results.

As you navigate the intricacies of macronutrient balance in your low-carb journey, consider this section your roadmap to crafting meals that not only align with your health goals but also tantalize your taste buds. Balancing proteins, fats, and carbohydrates strategically is the key to unlocking the full potential of a top Low Carb Diet Meal Plan, ensuring a delicious and nourishing experience with every bite.

Tailoring Your Meal Plan to Your Lifestyle

In the dynamic tapestry of our daily lives, a successful Low Carb Diet Meal Plan is one that seamlessly integrates into your unique lifestyle. In this section, we explore the art of tailoring your meal plan to suit your preferences, routines, and personal dietary needs, ensuring that the benefits of a low-carb lifestyle enhance rather than disrupt your daily existence.

Understanding Your Dietary Preferences

Every individual has distinct tastes and preferences when it comes to food. Whether you're a fan of savory dishes, have a sweet tooth, or crave variety in your meals, understanding your culinary inclinations forms the foundation of a meal plan that you'll genuinely enjoy. Discover how to adapt classic recipes or explore new culinary territories while staying true to your low-carb goals.

Adapting to Busy Schedules

For those with bustling schedules, meal prepping and planning become invaluable tools. Learn practical strategies to prepare and store low-carb meals in advance, ensuring that healthy options are readily available even on the busiest days. From quick and easy recipes to batch cooking, discover how to make your low-carb lifestyle a seamless part of your on-the-go routine.

Flexibility for Social Occasions

Social gatherings and events often revolve around food, and navigating these situations while adhering to a low-carb lifestyle can be a rewarding challenge. Gain insights into making mindful choices at restaurants, potlucks, and celebrations, allowing you to enjoy social occasions without compromising your dietary goals. Flexibility is the key to long-term success.

Accounting for Dietary Restrictions

Individuals with dietary restrictions, such as allergies or specific health conditions, may need to tailor their low-carb meal plans accordingly. Explore alternative ingredients, substitutes, and creative cooking techniques that cater to your unique dietary needs while ensuring your meals remain flavorful and satisfying.

Embracing Culinary Creativity

The journey of crafting a top Low Carb Diet Meal Plan is an opportunity to embrace culinary creativity. Experiment with a diverse array of low-carb ingredients, herbs, and spices. Discover how to turn simple, wholesome foods into culinary delights that cater to your taste buds and nutritional requirements.

As we navigate the process of tailoring your low-carb meal plan to your lifestyle, remember that flexibility, creativity, and understanding your unique preferences are essential components. This section serves as your guide to making the low-carb lifestyle not just a dietary choice but a sustainable and enjoyable aspect of your everyday life. Prepare to savor the benefits of a thoughtfully customized Low Carb Diet Meal Plan that harmonizes with your lifestyle, ensuring a journey towards a healthier and more vibrant you.

Chapter 4: Delicious Starch-Free Recipes

Welcome to the heart of your culinary adventure in Starch-Free Living. In this chapter, we embark on a journey through a collection of mouthwatering and nourishing Starch-Free recipes. Each dish is meticulously crafted to tantalize your taste buds while adhering to the principles of a starch-free lifestyle, proving that a diet focused on health can be both delectable and satisfying.

Breakfast Delights: Energizing Starch-Free Starters

Breakfast sets the tone for the day, and our Starch-Free recipes ensure a vibrant start. From fluffy omelets bursting with veggies to creative avocado-based delights, this section introduces you to a variety of breakfast options that not only energize your mornings but also align with your Starch-Free journey.

Lunchtime Pleasures: Satisfying Midday Starch-Free Meals

Lunch becomes a culinary celebration with a diverse array of Starch-Free options. Explore hearty salads featuring nutrient-rich greens, protein-packed main courses without the starch overload, and inventive wraps using alternatives like lettuce leaves. These recipes make midday meals not only satisfying but also a highlight of your Starch-Free day.

Dinner Triumphs: Flavorful Starch-Free Dinners

Dinner is transformed into a feast with our collection of Starch-Free recipes that redefine the evening meal. From succulent protein dishes paired with colorful vegetables to comforting soups and stews sans starch, this section guides you through creating dinners that are both indulgent and health-conscious.

Snack Attack: Guilt-Free Starch-Free Snacks

Snacking takes center stage in this section, where we present a variety of guilt-free, Starch-Free snack options. From crispy kale chips to protein-packed nut mixes, these snacks not only curb cravings but also contribute to your overall well-being, ensuring you stay satisfied between meals without compromising your Starch-Free commitment.

Sweet Endings: Desserts without the Starch

Cap off your Starch-Free day with a delightful array of desserts that prove you don't need starch to indulge in sweetness. From fruity delights to decadent chocolate treats, this section showcases desserts that not only satisfy your sweet tooth but also adhere to the principles of Starch-Free Living.

Each recipe in this chapter is a testament to the notion that Starch-Free Living doesn't mean sacrificing flavor or culinary joy. It's an invitation to explore the vast and delicious possibilities that align with your commitment to health. So, roll up your sleeves, gather your ingredients, and let's embark on a culinary journey that proves Starch-Free can be synonymous with scrumptious.

Breakfast Delights: Energizing Starch-Free Starters

Breakfast, often hailed as the most important meal of the day, takes center stage in our Starch-Free culinary adventure. Say goodbye to the monotony of traditional starch-laden breakfasts and embrace a world of energizing and flavorful Starch-Free starters that kickstart your day with vitality.

Fluffy Veggie Omelet

Indulge in the classic allure of a fluffy veggie omelet, where farm-fresh eggs envelop a colorful medley of bell peppers, tomatoes, spinach, and mushrooms. This protein-packed delight not only satisfies your morning hunger but also provides a burst of essential nutrients to fuel your day.

Avocado and Smoked Salmon Roll-Ups

Experience breakfast sophistication with Avocado and Smoked Salmon Roll-Ups – a harmonious blend of creamy avocado slices cradling savory smoked salmon. This elegant dish not only satisfies your taste buds but also delivers a dose of healthy fats and omega-3 fatty acids to kickstart your morning on a nutritious note.

Chia Seed Pudding Parfait

Delight your senses with a Chia Seed Pudding Parfait, where layers of chia seed pudding, fresh berries, and a sprinkle of nuts create a visually appealing and nutrient-dense breakfast. This Starch-Free alternative to traditional cereals is rich in fiber, antioxidants, and omega-3 fatty acids, offering a deliciously healthy way to begin your day.

Vegetable and Cheese Frittata Muffins

For those on the go, our Vegetable and Cheese Frittata Muffins are the perfect solution. Packed with sautéed vegetables and savory cheese, these grab-and-go delights make breakfast a breeze. Enjoy a protein-rich, Starch-Free option that suits your busy lifestyle without compromising on taste.

Zucchini and Egg Breakfast Pizza

Transform your morning routine with a Zucchini and Egg Breakfast Pizza, where thinly sliced zucchini forms the base for a flavorful combination of eggs, cheese, and your favorite herbs. This creative take on breakfast pizza proves that Starch-Free Living can be both imaginative and delicious.

These breakfast delights are just a glimpse into the flavorful possibilities that Starch-Free Living has to offer. With each energizing bite, you'll not only nourish your body but also set the tone for a day filled with vitality and satisfaction. Embrace the joy of Starch-Free breakfasts and savor the delicious journey toward a healthier and more vibrant you.

Lunchtime Pleasures: Satisfying Midday Starch-Free Meals

As the sun climbs in the sky, it's time to revel in the pleasure of Starch-Free lunches that not only satisfy your midday hunger but also elevate your culinary experience. Say goodbye to the heavy feeling that often accompanies starch-laden lunches and embrace a world of vibrant, satisfying Starch-Free midday delights.

Mediterranean Chicken Salad Bowl

Transport your taste buds to the Mediterranean with a refreshing Chicken Salad Bowl. Grilled chicken marinated in aromatic herbs meets a symphony of crisp cucumbers, cherry tomatoes, olives, and feta cheese. Drizzled with a light olive oil dressing, this Starch-Free creation is a tantalizing ode to freshness and flavor.

Cauliflower Fried Rice with Shrimp

Indulge in the savory delight of Cauliflower Fried Rice with Shrimp – a Starch-Free rendition of a classic favorite. Riced cauliflower takes center stage, mingling with succulent shrimp, colorful vegetables, and a hint of soy sauce. This wholesome dish proves that you can enjoy the comforting flavors of fried rice without the starch.

Grilled Veggie Wrap with Tofu

Elevate your lunchtime experience with a Grilled Veggie Wrap featuring tofu as the star. Vibrant, marinated vegetables encase grilled tofu, creating a satisfying and flavorful handheld delight. This Starch-Free wrap is not only a feast for the senses but also a wholesome and nutritious choice for your midday repast.

Salmon and Avocado Nori Rolls

Immerse yourself in the world of Japanese-inspired cuisine with Salmon and Avocado Nori Rolls. These delightful rolls feature fresh salmon, creamy avocado, and crisp vegetables wrapped in nori seaweed. Paired with a tangy dipping sauce, this Starch-Free creation adds a touch of elegance to your lunchtime routine.

Zesty Chickpea and Vegetable Stir-Fry

Experience the zing of a Zesty Chickpea and Vegetable Stir-Fry that brings together the goodness of chickpeas with a colorful array of stir-fried veggies. The combination of bold flavors and textures makes this Starch-Free dish a lunchtime favorite that satisfies both your palate and your nutritional needs.

These lunchtime pleasures are a testament to the diversity and satisfaction that Starch-Free Living can bring to your midday meals. Each bite is an opportunity to nourish your body with wholesome ingredients while savoring the delightful flavors of a Starch-Free culinary adventure. So, as the clock strikes noon, indulge in these satisfying Starch-Free meals that fuel your day with both pleasure and nutrition.

Dinner Triumphs: Flavorful Starch-Free Dinners

As the day winds down, embark on a journey through Flavorful Starch-Free Dinners that not only satiate your evening hunger but also transform your dinner table into a culinary celebration. Bid farewell to starch-heavy evening meals and relish the joy of wholesome, flavorful dishes that embrace the essence of Starch-Free Living.

Cauliflower and Broccoli Gratin

Elevate your dinner experience with a Cauliflower and Broccoli Gratin that redefines comfort food. Creamy cauliflower and broccoli florets are enveloped in a luscious cheese sauce and baked to perfection, creating a Starch-Free gratin that's both indulgent and wholesome.

Herb-Crusted Salmon with Roasted Vegetables

Immerse yourself in the delectable world of Herb-Crusted Salmon paired with Roasted Vegetables.

The salmon, adorned with a flavorful herb crust, takes center stage alongside a medley of oven-roasted vegetables. This Starch-Free dinner triumph is a testament to the marriage of simplicity and sophistication on your plate.

Zoodle Bolognese

Experience the Italian classic with a Starch-Free twist – Zoodle Bolognese. Spiraled zucchini noodles stand in for traditional pasta, serving as the perfect canvas for a rich and savory Bolognese sauce. This dish allows you to savor the essence of hearty Italian cuisine without the starch load.

Grilled Chicken and Vegetable Skewers

Embrace the simplicity of Grilled Chicken and Vegetable Skewers, where succulent chicken pieces are threaded onto skewers alongside vibrant vegetables. The marriage of grilled flavors and a zesty marinade creates a Starch-Free dinner that's both visually appealing and satisfying to the palate.

Eggplant Lasagna

Revel in the layers of flavor in a Starch-Free Eggplant Lasagna. Thin slices of eggplant take the place of traditional lasagna noodles, creating a delicious and hearty dish. With layers of marinara, cheese, and seasoned ground meat, this Eggplant Lasagna is a comforting Starch-Free alternative that doesn't compromise on taste.

These dinner triumphs are a testament to the rich and satisfying possibilities that Starch-Free Living brings to your evening meals. Each recipe is a celebration of flavors, textures, and nutritional goodness, proving that a Starch-Free dinner is not just a culinary choice but a delightful experience for your taste buds and well-being. As you gather around the dinner table, savor the joy of these Flavorful Starch-Free Dinners that transform every evening meal into a culinary masterpiece.

Snack Attack: Guilt-Free Starch-Free Snacks

Satisfy your cravings between meals with a collection of Guilt-Free Starch-Free Snacks that not only curb your hunger but also add a burst of flavor to your day. Say goodbye to mindless munching on starch-heavy treats and embrace a world of nutritious, delicious snacks designed to keep you energized and on track with your Starch-Free lifestyle.

Crispy Kale Chips

Indulge in the addictive crunch of Crispy Kale Chips – a nutrient-dense alternative to traditional potato chips. Lightly seasoned and oven-baked to perfection, these Starch-Free chips are not just a snack; they're a flavorful invitation to enjoy the goodness of leafy greens in every bite.

Protein-Packed Nut Mix

Elevate your snack game with a Protein-Packed Nut Mix that combines the satisfying crunch of almonds, walnuts, and cashews with the richness of dark chocolate or dried fruits. This Starch-Free snack not only provides a boost of energy but also delivers essential nutrients in a convenient, portable package.

Cheesy Zucchini Bites

Experience the savory delight of Cheesy Zucchini Bites – bite-sized morsels that pack a flavorful punch. Grated zucchini, combined with cheese and savory herbs, is baked to golden perfection, offering a Starch-Free snack that's both satisfying and delectable.

Avocado and Salsa Dip with Veggie Sticks

Dive into the creamy goodness of an Avocado and Salsa Dip paired with crisp Veggie Sticks. This refreshing and nutritious Starch-Free snack is a celebration of vibrant flavors, providing a perfect balance of creamy avocado and zesty salsa to tantalize your taste buds.

Spiced Chickpeas

Kick up the flavor with Spiced Chickpeas – a crunchy Starch-Free snack that marries the bold taste of chickpeas with a medley of spices. Whether roasted or air-fried, these flavorful chickpeas offer a satisfying and protein-rich option for your snack cravings.

These Guilt-Free Starch-Free Snacks are designed to prove that satisfying your snack cravings doesn't mean compromising your commitment to Starch-Free Living. Each bite is a step towards a healthier, more vibrant you. So, the next time the snack attack strikes, reach for these delightful Starch-Free options and savor the joy of guilt-free munching.

Sweet Endings: Desserts without the Starch

Indulge your sweet tooth without compromising your commitment to Starch-Free Living with a delightful array of Desserts without the Starch. From fruity delights to decadent chocolate treats, this section offers a collection of sweet endings that prove you can have your dessert and eat it too, even on a Starch-Free journey.

Berry Bliss Chia Pudding

Embark on a journey of Berry Bliss with a Chia Pudding that combines the richness of chia seeds with the sweetness of fresh berries. Layers of chia pudding and vibrant berries create a visually appealing and flavor-packed Starch-Free dessert that's as delightful to the eyes as it is to the palate.

Chocolate Avocado Mousse

Savor the decadence of a Chocolate Avocado Mousse that redefines the world of creamy desserts. Avocado, with its luscious texture, combines with rich cocoa to create a silky smooth mousse. This Starch-Free indulgence is not only a treat for your taste buds but also a celebration of nourishing ingredients.

Coconut and Berry Parfait

Elevate your dessert experience with a Coconut and Berry Parfait that layers coconut cream with fresh berries. The combination of creamy coconut and the burst of berry flavors offers a Starch-Free dessert that's both visually stunning and satisfying to the senses.

Almond Flour Lemon Bars

Treat yourself to the citrusy goodness of Almond Flour Lemon Bars – a Starch-Free alternative to the classic dessert. Almond flour forms the perfect crust for a zesty lemon filling, creating a delectable treat that showcases the bright and refreshing flavors of citrus without the starch content.

Vanilla Chia Seed Pudding with Cinnamon

Enjoy the timeless appeal of Vanilla Chia Seed Pudding with a hint of Cinnamon. This Starch-Free dessert offers a perfect balance of vanilla-infused chia pudding, topped with a sprinkle of cinnamon. It's a simple yet elegant way to conclude your meal on a sweet note.

These Sweet Endings without the Starch prove that Starch-Free Living doesn't mean bidding farewell to the joy of desserts. Each recipe in this section is a celebration of flavors, textures, and the art of crafting indulgent treats that align with your commitment to a Starch-Free lifestyle. So, as you embark on the journey of sweet endings, relish the delightful possibilities that await you in the world of Starch-Free desserts.

Chapter 5: Low-Carb Cookbook Extravaganza

Welcome to a culinary extravaganza that explores the rich tapestry of low-carb delights. In this chapter, we delve into a collection of recipes that not only adhere to the principles of a low-carb lifestyle but also celebrate the diverse and flavorful world of cuisine. From breakfast to dinner, snacks to desserts, this Low-Carb Cookbook Extravaganza is your passport to a culinary journey that proves low-carb can be both delicious and satisfying.

Rise and Shine: Low-Carb Breakfast Bliss

Embark on your day with a selection of Low-Carb Breakfast Bliss recipes that redefine the first meal of the day. From hearty omelets and innovative wraps to energizing smoothies, these breakfast options cater to a variety of tastes while keeping your carb intake in check.

Midday Delights: Low-Carb Lunchtime Feasts

Lunch becomes a celebration with a variety of Low-Carb Lunchtime Feasts that elevate midday meals to new heights. Explore vibrant salads, protein-packed main courses, and creative wraps that not only satisfy your hunger but also align with your commitment to a low-carb lifestyle.

Dinner Elegance: Low-Carb Culinary Creations

Transform your evenings with a selection of Low-Carb Culinary Creations that redefine dinner. From succulent grilled dishes and flavorful stir-fries to comforting casseroles, these recipes showcase the versatility and elegance that low-carb cooking can bring to your dinner table.

Snack Spectacle: Low-Carb Munching Mastery

Conquer your cravings with a Snack Spectacle that explores the realm of Low-Carb Munching Mastery. From crunchy nuts and savory dips to cheese platters and guilt-free treats, these low-carb snacks prove that satisfying your cravings doesn't mean compromising your dietary goals.

Sweet Sensations: Low-Carb Dessert Delights

Cap off your meals with a selection of Sweet Sensations that redefine dessert on a low-carb journey. Indulge in fruity parfaits, creamy mousses, and decadent treats that showcase the art of crafting desserts without the carb overload.

This Low-Carb Cookbook Extravaganza is more than just a collection of recipes; it's a testament to the richness and creativity that low-carb living can bring to your culinary experience. Each recipe is a celebration of flavors, textures, and the joy of savoring delicious meals while keeping your carb intake in check. So, immerse yourself in this extravaganza and discover the endless possibilities that await you on the journey of low-carb cooking.

Exploring the Low-Carb Culinary Universe

Prepare to embark on a culinary odyssey through the Low-Carb Culinary Universe, where dinner becomes a canvas for innovative and satisfying creations. In this section, we unravel the art of crafting Low-Carb Culinary Creations that redefine dinner with elegance, flavor, and wholesome goodness.

Grilled Salmon with Lemon-Dill Sauce

Elevate your evenings with the succulence of Grilled Salmon adorned with a zesty Lemon-Dill Sauce. The delicate balance of smoky grilled flavors and the bright citrusy notes creates a Low-Carb dinner masterpiece that is both nutritious and indulgent.

Cauliflower Fried Rice with Shrimp

Transport your taste buds to the heart of Asian cuisine with Cauliflower Fried Rice featuring succulent shrimp. Riced cauliflower takes center stage, absorbing the savory flavors of stir-fried vegetables and shrimp. This Low-Carb rendition of a classic dish proves that you can enjoy the essence of fried rice without the carb content.

Mediterranean Chicken Skewers with Tzatziki

Experience the flavors of the Mediterranean with Chicken Skewers paired with refreshing Tzatziki. Succulent chicken pieces, marinated in Mediterranean herbs and spices, are grilled to perfection and served with a cool and tangy Tzatziki sauce. This Low-Carb dish is a celebration of vibrant tastes and culinary elegance.

Zoodle Alfredo with Grilled Chicken

Indulge in the richness of Zoodle Alfredo with Grilled Chicken, where spiralized zucchini stands in for traditional pasta. Velvety Alfredo sauce, paired with grilled chicken, creates a Low-Carb pasta dish that's both comforting and guilt-free.

Stir-Fried Beef and Broccoli

Enter the realm of savory delights with Stir-Fried Beef and Broccoli – a classic Asian-inspired dish without the carb-heavy sauce. Tender strips of beef mingle with crisp broccoli in a savory stir-fry sauce, showcasing the mastery of low-carb cooking without sacrificing flavor.

These Low-Carb Culinary Creations are more than just dinner options; they're an exploration of the vast and delicious universe that low-carb living has to offer. As you savor each bite, revel in the joy of crafting elegant, flavorful, and health-conscious dinners that align with your commitment to a low-carb lifestyle. Welcome to the extraordinary world of the Low-Carb Culinary Universe, where every dinner is a masterpiece waiting to be savored.

Low-Carb Delicacies for Every Palate

Dive into the enchanting realm of Low-Carb Delicacies that cater to every palate. In this section, we unveil a collection of dinner recipes designed to captivate your taste buds with an array of flavors, textures, and culinary ingenuity. From savory grilled dishes to comforting stir-fries, these Low-Carb creations ensure that every dinner is a journey of delight for every discerning palate.

Zesty Lemon Garlic Shrimp Skewers

Embark on a flavor-packed journey with Zesty Lemon Garlic Shrimp Skewers that bring the taste of the sea to your dinner table. Succulent shrimp marinated in a zesty blend of lemon, garlic, and herbs are threaded onto skewers and grilled to perfection. This Low-Carb dish is a symphony of freshness and bold Mediterranean flavors.

Spaghetti Squash Primavera

Experience the joy of Italian cuisine with a Low-Carb twist – Spaghetti Squash Primavera. Delicate strands of roasted spaghetti squash become the canvas for a colorful medley of seasonal vegetables and a light, herb-infused sauce. This dish showcases the art of transforming vegetables into a satisfying and flavorful pasta alternative.

Stuffed Bell Peppers with Turkey and Cauliflower Rice

Elevate your dinner table with Stuffed Bell Peppers featuring a wholesome filling of lean turkey and cauliflower rice. Each vibrant bell pepper becomes a vessel for a savory and protein-packed delight. This Low-Carb creation is not just a feast for the eyes but also a nourishing option for those seeking a comforting and health-conscious dinner.

Cajun Chicken and Sausage Skillet

Ignite your taste buds with the bold flavors of a Cajun Chicken and Sausage Skillet. Juicy chicken, savory sausage, and a medley of vegetables are expertly seasoned with Cajun spices, creating a one-pan wonder that's both convenient and explosively flavorful. This Low-Carb dish promises a culinary journey through the vibrant landscape of Cajun cuisine.

Greek Salad with Grilled Lamb

Transport yourself to the sun-kissed shores of Greece with a refreshing Greek Salad paired with Grilled Lamb. Crisp cucumbers, tomatoes, olives, and feta cheese mingle with perfectly grilled lamb, creating a Low-Carb masterpiece that combines the essence of a Greek salad with the savory satisfaction of grilled meat.

These Low-Carb Delicacies are a testament to the culinary diversity that low-carb living offers. As you savor these dinner options, relish the satisfaction of crafting meals that not only cater to your dietary goals but also celebrate the rich tapestry of flavors. Whether you crave the freshness of seafood, the warmth of Italian-inspired dishes, or the bold spices of Cajun cuisine, these Low-Carb Delicacies promise an exquisite dining experience for every palate.

Mastering Low-Carb Cooking Techniques

Embark on a journey of culinary mastery as we delve into the art and science of Low-Carb Cooking Techniques. In this section, we explore the principles and methods that form the foundation of crafting delicious, health-conscious meals without compromising on flavor. Whether you're a seasoned chef or a kitchen novice, these techniques will empower you to elevate your low-carb cooking to new heights.

Understanding Substitutes and Alternatives

Discover the world of substitutes and alternatives that make low-carb cooking both creative and satisfying. From cauliflower rice to zucchini noodles, explore how these versatile ingredients can replace traditional high-carb elements, transforming classic dishes into low-carb delights without sacrificing taste.

Mastering Low-Carb Sauces and Seasonings

Unlock the secrets of crafting flavorful sauces and seasonings that enhance the taste of your low-carb creations. Learn to balance herbs, spices, and other aromatics to create mouthwatering blends that elevate your dishes. From simple vinaigrettes to complex marinades, these techniques will become your passport to a world of sensational low-carb flavors.

Grilling and Roasting Techniques for Low-Carb Success

Explore the nuances of grilling and roasting to bring out the natural flavors of your ingredients. From perfectly grilled proteins to roasted vegetables with caramelized edges, these techniques add depth and richness to your low-carb meals. Master the art of temperature control and seasoning to create dishes that are not just low in carbs but high in culinary excellence.

Low-Carb Baking Without Compromise

Delve into the realm of low-carb baking without compromising on taste and texture. Learn to use almond flour, coconut flour, and other low-carb alternatives to create baked goods that are not only delicious but also align with your dietary goals. From bread to desserts, these baking techniques ensure that you can enjoy the pleasures of the oven without the carb overload.

Innovative Meal Prep for Low-Carb Success

Efficiency meets excellence with innovative meal prep techniques designed for low-carb success. Discover how to streamline your cooking process, plan ahead, and create batches of low-carb meals that suit your lifestyle. These meal prep strategies ensure that you always have nutritious and delicious options on hand, making low-carb living a seamless part of your routine.

As you delve into mastering these Low-Carb Cooking Techniques, consider this section your culinary toolkit for crafting meals that are not only low in carbs but also high in flavor and satisfaction. Whether you're experimenting with substitutes, perfecting your grilling skills, or diving into the world of low-carb baking, these techniques will empower you to create a diverse and delightful array of low-carb dishes. Welcome to the art of mastering low-carb cooking—a journey that transforms every meal into a masterpiece of health-conscious culinary brilliance.

Chapter 6: Putting It All Together

In the grand finale of our culinary journey, we bring together the wisdom and recipes from the previous chapters, guiding you in seamlessly incorporating the Complete Starch Solution Diet and Low-Carb Cookbook Extravaganza into your daily life. This chapter is a roadmap for translating knowledge into action, ensuring that the principles and flavors explored throughout this book become a natural and sustainable part of your lifestyle.

Crafting Your Personalized Meal Plan

As you embark on your journey to embrace Starch-Free Living and Low-Carb Delicacies, it's time to craft a personalized meal plan tailored to your tastes, preferences, and lifestyle. Learn how to create a week's worth of meals that not only align with your dietary goals but also delight your taste buds. From breakfast to dinner, snacks to desserts, discover the art of designing a meal plan that nourishes both body and soul.

Efficient Meal Prep Strategies

Efficiency is the key to success, especially when adopting a new way of eating. Uncover time-saving and efficient meal prep strategies that allow you to stay on track with your Starch-Free and Low-Carb lifestyle, even on the busiest days. Whether you're a busy professional, a parent on the go, or simply someone seeking convenience, these strategies ensure that nutritious and delicious meals are always within reach.

Navigating Social Settings and Dining Out

Social occasions and dining out can present unique challenges, but they don't have to derail your Starch-Free and Low-Carb journey. Gain insights into navigating diverse social settings, making mindful choices at restaurants, and enjoying celebrations without compromising your dietary goals. With a few thoughtful strategies, you can confidently embrace your lifestyle choices while savoring the joy of communal dining.

Embracing Long-Term Success

Success in adopting the Complete Starch Solution Diet and Low-Carb lifestyle isn't just about short-term changes; it's about creating sustainable habits for long-term well-being. Explore tips and practices that support your ongoing journey, from staying motivated to adjusting your approach as needed. Discover how to make Starch-Free Living and Low-Carb cooking not just a phase but a lifelong celebration of health and culinary joy.

Continuing Your Culinary Adventure

As you reach the conclusion of this book, consider it not an endpoint but a stepping stone in your culinary adventure. Continue to explore new recipes, refine your cooking skills, and stay attuned to the evolving landscape of Starch-Free and Low-Carb living. This chapter provides a launchpad for your ongoing journey, encouraging you to discover, create, and savor the richness that a health-conscious and flavorful lifestyle can offer.

In Putting It All Together, we empower you to transform knowledge into practice, ensuring that the principles and recipes shared throughout this book become an integral part of your daily routine. This chapter marks the beginning of a new chapter in your culinary journey—one where Starch-Free Living and Low-Carb delights seamlessly weave into the fabric of your vibrant and health-conscious lifestyle. Cheers to a future filled with delicious possibilities and sustained well-being!

Week-by-Week Starch-Free Meal Plans

Welcome to the practical guide on crafting Week-by Week Starch-Free Meal Plans. In this section, we'll break down the process of translating the principles of the Complete Starch Solution Diet into tangible, delicious meals that form the foundation of your Starch-Free lifestyle. Follow along as we design a week's worth of balanced and flavorful

Starch-Free meal plans that cater to your nutritional needs and culinary preferences.

Week 1: The Foundation

Dive into the Starch-Free lifestyle with a foundational week that introduces you to the key elements of Starch-Free Living. Enjoy energizing breakfasts, satisfying lunches, and flavorful dinners that showcase the diversity and vibrancy of meals without starch. From vegetable omelets to grilled protein dishes, Week 1 sets the stage for a delicious journey ahead.

Week 2: Exploring Variety

Expand your culinary horizons in Week 2 by exploring a wider range of Starch-Free options. Experiment with different vegetables, proteins, and cooking methods to add variety to your meals. From creative salads to inventive wraps, this week invites you to savor the richness of Starch-Free living with a newfound sense of culinary adventure.

Week 3: Flavorful Discoveries

Embark on Week 3 with a focus on Flavorful Discoveries. Delve into diverse herbs, spices, and seasonings to enhance the taste of your Starch-Free creations. Whether it's a zesty marinade for grilled dishes or a refreshing dressing for salads, this week encourages you to play with flavors, making each meal a delightful and satisfying experience.

Week 4: Nourishing Wellness

As you enter Week 4, prioritize Nourishing Wellness by incorporating nutrient-dense ingredients that support your overall well-being. Explore recipes rich in vitamins, minerals, and essential nutrients, ensuring that your Starch-Free journey is not only delicious but also a source of holistic nourishment.

Week 5: Customizing for Lifestyle

Tailor your Starch-Free Meal Plans to your lifestyle needs in Week 5. Whether you're a busy professional, a fitness enthusiast, or someone with specific dietary requirements, this week provides insights into customizing your meals for optimal energy, performance, and satisfaction. Discover the art of making Starch-Free living seamlessly fit into your daily routine.

Week 6: Celebration of Success

Cap off your six-week journey with a Celebration of Success in Week 6. Reflect on the positive changes, culinary discoveries, and newfound well-being that Starch-Free Living has brought to your life. Enjoy indulgent yet health-conscious meals that celebrate your commitment to long-term success, creating a joyful conclusion to this transformative culinary adventure.

By the end of this section, you'll not only have a comprehensive Week-by-Week Starch-Free Meal Plan but also the knowledge and confidence to continue crafting your own delicious and health-conscious menus. Embrace the richness of Starch-Free Living as a sustainable lifestyle, and may each week be a celebration of culinary joy, well-being, and continued success on your Starch-Free journey.

Staying Committed: Tips for Long-Term Success

As you embark on the journey of Starch-Free Living and embrace the principles outlined in this cookbook, sustaining long-term success becomes paramount. In this section, we provide valuable insights and practical tips to help you stay committed to your health-conscious lifestyle. From maintaining motivation to navigating challenges, these strategies will empower you to make Starch-Free Living a sustainable and rewarding part of your daily routine.

1. Set Realistic Goals: Begin by setting achievable and realistic goals. Whether it's incorporating more Starch-Free meals into your week or gradually reducing starch intake, establishing tangible objectives will keep you motivated and focused on your long-term journey.

2. Embrace Variety: Keep your Starch-Free lifestyle exciting by embracing variety. Experiment with different vegetables, proteins, and cooking techniques to prevent monotony and ensure a diverse range of nutrients in your meals. Variety not only enhances the dining experience but also contributes to a well-rounded nutritional profile.

3. Plan and Prep: Planning and meal preparation are essential for success. Dedicate time each week to plan your meals, create shopping lists, and prep ingredients. Having Starch-Free options readily available reduces the likelihood of succumbing to convenience foods that may not align with your dietary goals.

4. Stay Educated: Stay informed about the benefits of Starch-Free Living and its impact on your health. Understanding the positive changes occurring in your body can be a powerful motivator.

Continuously educate yourself on new recipes, ingredients, and cooking techniques to keep the journey fresh and inspiring.

5. Celebrate Milestones: Acknowledge and celebrate your achievements along the way. Whether it's a month of consistent Starch-Free meals or successfully navigating a social event while adhering to your dietary choices, each milestone is a testament to your commitment. Reward yourself with non-food treats to reinforce positive behavior.

6. Build a Support System: Surround yourself with a supportive community. Share your Starch-Free journey with friends, family, or online communities who understand and encourage your choices. Having a support system provides motivation, accountability, and a sense of connection on your health-conscious path.

7. Listen to Your Body: Pay attention to how your body responds to Starch-Free Living. Notice changes in energy levels, digestion, and overall well-being. Your body's signals are valuable feedback, helping you tailor your Starch-Free lifestyle to suit your unique needs and preferences.

8. Navigate Challenges Mindfully: Challenges may arise, but mindfulness is your ally. Whether faced with social settings, travel, or unexpected cravings, approach challenges with awareness. Develop strategies to navigate these situations without compromising your commitment to Starch-Free Living.

9. Adapt and Evolve: Recognize that your Starch-Free journey is dynamic and may require adaptation. As your tastes, lifestyle, and health goals evolve, be open to adjusting your approach. Flexibility and adaptability ensure that your Starch-Free lifestyle remains a positive and sustainable choice.

10. Seek Professional Guidance: If needed, seek guidance from healthcare professionals or nutritionists familiar with Starch-Free diets. They can provide personalized advice, address concerns, and offer tailored recommendations to support your health goals.

By integrating these tips into your lifestyle, you can foster a sense of empowerment and resilience on your Starch-Free journey. Staying committed to long-term success is not just about dietary choices; it's a holistic approach that encompasses mindfulness, celebration, and ongoing self-discovery. May each day be a step forward on your path to sustained well-being through Starch-Free Living.

Celebrating Your Starch-Free Journey

As you reach the culmination of this transformative experience, it's time to celebrate the milestones, discoveries, and positive changes that your Starch-Free journey has brought to your life. In this section, we explore the importance of recognizing and commemorating your achievements, making the celebration an integral part of your ongoing commitment to Starch-Free Living.

1. Reflect on Achievements: Take a moment to reflect on the achievements you've made during your Starch-Free journey. Whether it's adapting to new cooking techniques, discovering flavorful recipes, or consistently choosing Starch-Free options, each accomplishment is a testament to your dedication and growth.

2. Create a Culinary Scrapbook: Document your favorite Starch-Free recipes, memorable meals, and culinary experiments in a dedicated culinary scrapbook. This not only serves as a visual celebration of your journey but also becomes a personalized cookbook filled with the flavors and memories of your Starch-Free lifestyle.

3. Host a Starch-Free Feast: Gather friends and family to share in the joy of your Starch-Free achievements by hosting a Starch-Free feast. Showcase your favorite recipes, introduce loved ones to the delicious world of Starch-Free Living, and create an atmosphere of celebration around health-conscious choices.

4. Acknowledge Mindful Eating: Celebrate the shift towards mindful eating that comes with Starch-Free Living. Appreciate the flavors, textures, and nourishment of each meal. Mindful eating not only enhances the dining experience but also fosters a deeper connection with the food you consume.

5. Reward Yourself: Treat yourself to a meaningful reward that aligns with your health-conscious goals. Whether it's a spa day, a new kitchen gadget, or an outdoor adventure, choose a reward that acknowledges your dedication to Starch-Free Living and motivates you to continue the journey.

6. Share Your Story: Inspire others by sharing your Starch-Free journey. Write a blog, contribute to online communities, or simply have conversations with friends and family about your experiences. Your story can be a source of motivation and support for others considering or undergoing a similar transformation.

7. Create a Wellness Ritual: Develop a wellness ritual that symbolizes the positive changes in your life. This could be a morning meditation, an evening walk, or any practice that fosters a sense of well-being. Let this ritual serve as a daily reminder of the balance and vitality that Starch-Free Living brings.

8. Express Gratitude: Express gratitude for the nourishment, vitality, and joy that Starch-Free Living has infused into your life. Acknowledge the positive impact on your health, energy levels, and overall well-being. Gratitude enhances the sense of fulfillment and reinforces the significance of your journey.

9. Set New Culinary Goals: Embrace the future with excitement by setting new culinary goals within the realm of Starch-Free Living. Whether it's mastering a challenging recipe, exploring a specific cuisine, or incorporating more plant-based options, these goals continue to fuel your culinary adventure.

10. Celebrate Each Day: Finally, celebrate each day as a unique opportunity to nourish your body, expand your culinary horizons, and savor the joy of Starch-Free Living. Let each meal be a celebration of your commitment to a health-conscious and flavorful lifestyle.

May the celebration of your Starch-Free journey be as vibrant and enriching as the journey itself. As you revel in the accomplishments and lessons learned, remember that celebrating is not just an endpoint but a continuous affirmation of your commitment to well-being. Cheers to a life filled with delicious possibilities, sustained health, and the ongoing joy of your Starch-Free adventure!

breakfast recipe and a dinner recipe

Ingredients:
- 4 large eggs
- 1 cup zucchini, grated
- 1 cup fresh spinach, chopped
- 1/2 cup cherry tomatoes, halved

- 1/4 cup feta cheese, crumbled

- 1 tablespoon olive oil

- Salt and pepper to taste

- Fresh herbs for garnish (e.g., parsley or chives)

Instructions:

1. Preheat the oven to 350°F (180°C).

2. In a bowl, whisk the eggs until well beaten. Season with salt and pepper.

3. Heat olive oil in an oven-safe skillet over medium heat.

4. Add grated zucchini to the skillet and cook for 2-3 minutes until softened.

5. Add chopped spinach and cherry tomatoes to the skillet. Cook for an additional 2 minutes until the spinach wilts.

6. Pour the beaten eggs over the vegetables in the skillet.

7. Sprinkle crumbled feta cheese evenly over the eggs.

8. Allow the edges to set for a minute, then transfer the skillet to the preheated oven.

9. Bake for 12-15 minutes or until the frittata is set and slightly golden.

10. Remove from the oven, let it cool for a few minutes, garnish with fresh herbs, slice, and serve.

Dinner Triumph: Grilled Lemon Herb Chicken with Asparagus

Ingredients:
- 4 boneless, skinless chicken breasts
- 1 bunch fresh asparagus, trimmed
- 3 tablespoons olive oil
- 2 cloves garlic, minced
- Zest and juice of 1 lemon
- 1 teaspoon dried oregano
- 1 teaspoon dried thyme
- Salt and pepper to taste
- Fresh parsley for garnish

Instructions:
1. Preheat the grill to medium-high heat.
2. In a small bowl, whisk together olive oil, minced garlic, lemon zest, lemon juice, oregano, thyme, salt, and pepper.
3. Place chicken breasts and trimmed asparagus on a baking sheet.

4. Brush the chicken breasts and asparagus with the prepared lemon herb marinade.

5. Grill the chicken for 6-7 minutes per side or until the internal temperature reaches 165°F (74°C).

6. Grill the asparagus for 4-5 minutes, turning occasionally until tender and slightly charred.

7. Remove the chicken and asparagus from the grill and let them rest for a few minutes.

8. Garnish with fresh parsley, serve, and enjoy your Starch-Free dinner delight!

Feel free to customize these recipes to suit your taste preferences and dietary needs. Happy cooking!

Avocado and shrimp salad

Ingredients:

- 1 lb (450g) shrimp, peeled and deveined

- 2 avocados, diced

- 1 cup cherry tomatoes, halved

- 1 cucumber, diced

- 1/4 cup red onion, finely chopped

- 1/4 cup fresh cilantro, chopped

- Juice of 2 limes
- 2 tablespoons olive oil
- Salt and pepper to taste
- Mixed greens for serving

Instructions:

1. In a large bowl, combine shrimp, diced avocados, cherry tomatoes, cucumber, red onion, and cilantro.

2. In a small bowl, whisk together lime juice, olive oil, salt, and pepper to create the dressing.

3. Pour the dressing over the shrimp and avocado mixture, gently tossing to coat evenly.

4. Refrigerate for at least 30 minutes to let the flavors meld.

5. Serve the avocado and shrimp salad over a bed of mixed greens, and enjoy a refreshing and satisfying Starch-Free lunch.

Snack Attack: Parmesan Zucchini Chips

Ingredients:

- 2 medium zucchinis, thinly sliced
- 1/2 cup grated Parmesan cheese

- 1 teaspoon garlic powder

- 1 teaspoon dried oregano

- Salt and pepper to taste

- Olive oil spray

Instructions:

1. Preheat your oven to 425°F (220°C) and line a baking sheet with parchment paper.

2. In a bowl, combine Parmesan cheese, garlic powder, dried oregano, salt, and pepper.

3. Lightly spray the zucchini slices with olive oil.

4. Dip each zucchini slice into the Parmesan mixture, coating both sides, and place them on the prepared baking sheet.

5. Bake for 15-20 minutes or until the zucchini chips are golden and crisp.

6. Allow the chips to cool for a few minutes before serving.

7. Enjoy these crispy Parmesan Zucchini Chips as a guilt-free Starch-Free snack.

Feel free to incorporate these recipes into your Starch-Free meal plans and share the delightful flavors with those around you. Happy cooking!

Absolutely! Here are a couple more delicious and Starch-Free recipes to add to your collection.

Cauliflower and Broccoli Gratin

Ingredients:

- 1 medium cauliflower, cut into florets

- 1 bunch broccoli, cut into florets

- 2 cups shredded cheddar cheese

- 1 cup heavy cream

- 2 cloves garlic, minced

- 1 teaspoon Dijon mustard

- Salt and pepper to taste

- 1/2 cup grated Parmesan cheese

- Fresh parsley for garnish

Instructions:

1. Preheat your oven to 375°F (190°C) and grease a baking dish.

2. Steam cauliflower and broccoli until just tender. Place them in the prepared baking dish.

3. In a saucepan over medium heat, combine shredded cheddar, heavy cream, minced garlic, Dijon mustard, salt, and pepper. Stir until the cheese is melted and the sauce is smooth.

4. Pour the cheese sauce over the cauliflower and broccoli, ensuring they are well coated.

5. Sprinkle grated Parmesan on top and bake for 20-25 minutes or until the gratin is bubbly and golden.

6. Garnish with fresh parsley before serving. Enjoy this comforting Starch-Free dinner delight.

Sweet Endings: Berry and Coconut Chia Pudding

Ingredients:

- 1/4 cup chia seeds

- 1 cup coconut milk

- 1 teaspoon vanilla extract

- 1 tablespoon maple syrup or sweetener of choice

- Mixed berries for topping (strawberries, blueberries, raspberries)

- Shredded coconut for garnish

Instructions:

1. In a bowl, mix chia seeds, coconut milk, vanilla extract, and maple syrup. Stir well to combine.

2. Cover the bowl and refrigerate for at least 2 hours or overnight, allowing the chia seeds to absorb the liquid and create a pudding-like consistency.

3. Before serving, give the chia pudding a good stir.

4. Spoon the chia pudding into serving glasses or bowls.

5. Top with a generous amount of mixed berries and a sprinkle of shredded coconut.

6. Serve chilled and savor this Starch-Free dessert that's both wholesome and indulgent.

These recipes bring a variety of flavors to your Starch-Free culinary journey. Feel free to experiment with ingredients and make these dishes your own! Enjoy your Starch-Free cooking adventure!

Conclusion

In the end, as Emily's journey unfolded within the pages of "The Complete Starch Solution Diet Cookbook Recipes," it became clear that the power of knowledge and its practical application had the ability to shape lives. The cookbook, once a simple purchase, became a catalyst for positive change, not only for Emily but for an entire community.

The transformative nature of the Complete Starch Solution Diet reached far beyond the boundaries of Emily's kitchen. As she shared her newfound culinary wisdom through workshops and community events, the ripple effect of healthy living spread, touching the lives of those eager to embrace a plant-based lifestyle. The cookbook, with its carefully curated recipes and nutritional guidance, served as a compass, leading individuals toward a healthier and more fulfilling way of life.

The community in Culinary Haven flourished, fueled by the shared passion for wholesome, plant-based meals. Emily's story became an inspiration, a testament to the impact that a single book could have on an individual's well-being and the collective health of a community.

As the final chapters of Emily's story unfolded, it became evident that the Complete Starch Solution Diet Cookbook was not just a compilation of recipes; it was a guide to a holistic and sustainable approach to nutrition. It empowered individuals to make informed choices, fostering a sense of responsibility for their own health and the well-being of those around them.

"The Complete Starch Solution Diet Cookbook Recipes" was not just a book on a shelf; it was a catalyst for positive change, a source of inspiration that transformed lives one meal at a time. Emily's journey underscored the profound impact that the right knowledge, coupled with action, could have on personal well-being and the wider community. In the world of Culinary Haven, the cookbook became a beacon of health, radiating the joy of nourishing both body and soul through the simple act of preparing a good, wholesome meal.